The Basic Principles of the Kelee®

A Step-by-Step Guide to Kelee Meditation

The Kelee Foundation

Ron W. Rathbun, Founder

Foreword by Daniel Lee, MD

THE BASIC PRINCIPLES OF THE KELEE®
A Step-by-Step Guide to Kelee Meditation

This book is an original publication of the Kelee Foundation

PRINTING HISTORY
First edition June 2013

www.thekelee.org

ISBN: 978-0-9893432-1-3

PRINTED IN THE UNITED STATES OF AMERICA

Acknowledgements

There are many people I would like to thank...

My mentor, Dr. Eugene C. Larr, who introduced me to the Kelee in 1985 and who I consulted with as new discoveries of the Kelee came to light.

Lavana Rathbun, CFO of the Kelee Foundation, for her support, patience, and love over the years as each day unfolded into the next.

Nikki Feldman, MBA, for all of her diligence and behind-the-scenes efforts in laying the groundwork of the Kelee Foundation, Quiescence Publishing, and the medical study.

Dr. Daniel Lee for starting the medical study at the University of California, San Diego Medical Center and for being open to seeing how profound and invaluable the knowledge of the Kelee is to medicine.

Dr. Amy Sitapati for her innate awareness of the Kelee, its importance, and her willingness to help bring the medical study about.

Frank Silva, MPH, for his input on this book and eagerness to teach the Practice.

Moira Mar-Tang, MPH, for the countless hours she has donated to help with the medical study.

There are many others who have freely offered their time and energy because they know it is important to the future of our planet to understand the difference between brain and mind.

If you want to heal yourself,

you have to feel good about yourself.

Why create or accept something that hurts you.

Solve these two equations and you will heal.

—*Ron W. Rathbun*

Contents

The feeling in our mind feeds the feeling in our body.
When our mind is growing and learning,
it is that feeling that manifests health and healing.

—*Ron W. Rathbun*

Foreword

By Daniel Lee, MD

So why should I do Kelee meditation? This is a question you are probably asking yourself and one that I posed to myself almost two and a half years ago. Interestingly, I was first introduced to Kelee meditation years prior to when I actually started in December of 2005. However, I did not have the motivation to start. Instead, I created many excuses why I could not meditate twice a day for five to ten minutes. It seemed interesting, but my life was good enough—or so it seemed. Why did I need to try this particular meditation practice?

Well, it turns out that life always seems to throw you a curve ball when you least expect. An unexpected breakup in my relationship occurred and I was devastated. The experience of emotional pain and constant negative thoughts about myself was the impetus for me to want to change.

I started Kelee meditation and was amazed at how doing it helped me to calm my negative thoughts over the initial six months. After all, I had been through other breakups in the past, but the pain and negativity seemed to last years. Kelee meditation helped me to learn more about myself through troubleshooting my own mind. Why did I take in and accept these negative thoughts and feelings as being true reflections of myself? Initially, the effects of Kelee meditation are subtle, but the insights and perceptions about yourself and how you relate with others become more apparent and profound with continued practice, persistence, and patience.

As I had personally seen and experienced the true changes within myself, I decided to offer my patients the opportunity to learn about this practice. Working with human immunodeficiency virus infected patients in my medical practice, I saw an excellent opportunity to help many of my patients who are living with a chronic illness. Furthermore, having this diagnosis can certainly worsen one's depression, anxiety, and stress levels. Many of my patients who have started Kelee meditation and remained consistent with it have noticed dramatic improvements in their quality of life. Many have told me how their usually persistent negative thoughts and feelings have calmed down over time. In addition, things (people or situations) that used to bother them don't bother them anymore. Ultimately, this is the hallmark of Kelee meditation.

To confirm these findings scientifically, I have just started a study to evaluate the effects of Kelee meditation on stress, anxiety, and depression and I have no doubt that improvements will be significant.

Thinking back, I often wonder why I was so reluctant to start this practice. My first excuse was that, "I don't have time to meditate." Kelee meditation only takes five to ten minutes twice per day. This is really time efficient when compared to other types of meditation, which may require up to half to one hour to perform. My second excuse was, "Why do I need to change my life if everything is fine?" In retrospect, it is clear to me now that I was deluding myself.

I believe that most people are "happy" with their lives, but do not realize that being able to free yourself from your own pain (without the use of medications or drugs), you can actually improve your own quality of life. It certainly has done that for my patients and for me. Who doesn't want to feel better?

I have often pondered why I had to wait for pain and suffering to occur before wanting to seek improvements in my life. I could have easily avoided some of the seemingly unnecessary suffering if I'd had a better understanding of why people or experiences in life cause me pain, an understanding which occurs over time through performing Kelee meditation.

Ron W. Rathbun has spent over twenty years working on understanding the Kelee and confirming his own findings in himself and in the many students he has taught over the years. He has now chosen to introduce the Kelee to the rest of the world as a means for people to free themselves from pain. The following pages outline the intellectual understanding of the Kelee—from how to do the meditation practice to how stillness of the mind leads to the harmonious effects of Kelee meditation. However, life is about experience—not just intellectual knowledge. Try this practice for yourself and truly experience life.

As a physician, I firmly believe that Kelee meditation has broad, countless applications in the medical field, as well as in all other aspects of life. Imagine proactively improving overall well-being by truly alleviating depression, anxiety, and stress without the use of medications. Reducing stress through Kelee meditation may lead people away from seeking social habits (smoking, drinking alcohol excessively, illicit drug use) to try to cope with the stressors of life. Imagine the impact that decreasing these psychological issues can have on the prevention of downstream medical consequences/conditions, such as hypertension, heart disease, and cancer. Imagine the potential cost savings on health care utilization that can be achieved by using Kelee meditation as preventative health care. Just imagine!

Ron W. Rathbun's Kelee meditation has certainly transformed my life and the way I think and feel about my life. Once you've experienced this for yourself, you will glimpse an understanding of the enormous, unlimited potential of what this practice can do for you. So what do you have to lose by trying this practice? Just negativity and discontentment. But don't take my word for it! Experience your own Kelee and then you will know for yourself what you have found—your true spiritual nature.

Daniel Lee, MD
Clinical Professor of Medicine
UCSD School of Medicine
UCSD Medical Center—Owen Clinic

If you are not paying attention
to your health,
who is responsible for it?

—*Ron W. Rathbun*

Introduction

Kelee meditation was founded after over two decades of research by a process of observing what works. It is not a theory; it is an understanding of the mind and simply put, it is the way it is. The basic principles in this book are all you need to get started to heal yourself on psychological and physiological levels. There is nothing in the physical body that the mind does not control. What can you do without your mind?

Have you ever noticed that when you feel bad mentally, you never feel good physically? This is because the mind runs the central nervous system, which runs the physical body. Everyone at one time or another has had a negative thought that upset his or her stomach. This is an example of when psychology has affected the physiology of the body. If negative thoughts are allowed to remain internalized permanently, physical problems manifest.

When the central nervous system and the cardiovascular system are stressed to constriction, major health problems occur over time. Doing Kelee meditation reverses the effects of stress by dissolving negative thought-form images in the mind, thus calming the central nervous system and the cardiovascular system at the same time. As you practice Kelee meditation, mental strength and harmony of mind develop over time. It is harmony of mind that boosts the immune system and healing rates in the physical body.

—Ron W. Rathbun, founder of Kelee meditation

Basic Principles
of the Kelee Defined

The Conscious Awareness: a point of perception between the intellectual outside physical world and the inside world of emotion.

Brain Function: thinks, analyzes, stores intellectual knowledge, and runs the physical body.

Mind Function: mentally feels or senses as an objective observer and is synonymous with a relaxed sense of perception; thus mind function leads into deeper states of awareness and innate knowing.

The Surface of the Mind: a horizontal plane of electrochemical energy at eye level. A division point between the brain (or intellect) and deeper states of mind. These states are associated with inner contentment and an overall sense of calm.

Lesser Kelee: an electrochemical field of energy above the surface of the mind that moves out laterally from the center, up over the top of the brain, then down in between both hemispheres of the brain, and folds into the brain network. The energy in the lesser Kelee has to do with how one relates to the outside physical world—people, places, and things.

Greater Kelee: an electrochemical field of energy that flows below the surface of the mind, down to about where one's heart is and then turns upward to join the lesser Kelee at the surface of the mind. The energy in the greater Kelee has to do with how one feels about oneself on an emotional level. The energy of the greater Kelee is related to matters of the heart (i.e., caring, kindness, and gentleness).

Compartments: synonymous with "baggage," emotional "buttons," or "issues" manifesting as nonproductive, inefficient behavioral traits.

Looping: occurs when one's conscious awareness is attached to a negative compartment, resulting in a repetitive circulation of destructive thoughts.

Detachment from Internal Compartments: the space within one's Kelee, where one lives when one is unaffected by negative thoughts and emotions.

Processing of Compartments: the means by which internalized electrochemical negativity dissipates and dissolves. A result of relaxing one's conscious awareness, stilling one's mind, and detaching from compartments.

The Flow of the Kelee: when the electrochemical energy of how one thinks and the energy of how one feels flow together in unison without beginning or end. Within the flow of the Kelee is a single point of perception known as the conscious awareness.

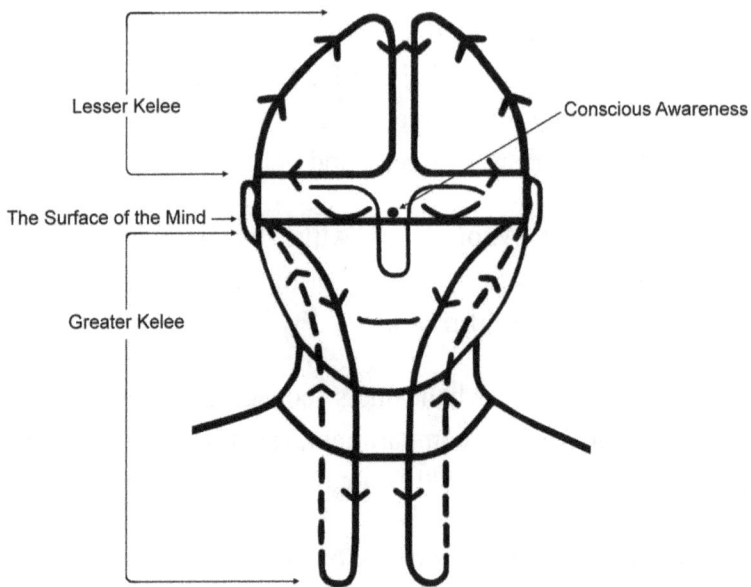

Lesser Kelee

Conscious Awareness

The Surface of the Mind →

Greater Kelee

Kelee Meditation

Step One: *Approximately two minutes.*

Sit down, get comfortable, and begin relaxing brain activity. Mentally feel the conscious awareness at the top of the head and mentally relax this horizontal plane of awareness through both hemispheres of the brain, ultimately settling at the surface of the mind. At the surface of the mind, be consciously relaxed, but not thinking.

Step Two: *Approximately three minutes.*

After relaxing at the surface of the mind, mentally allow the conscious awareness to drop below the surface of the mind, to a still point within the greater Kelee. The goal is to let go of sense consciousness and experience total stillness for about three minutes.

Note: Before dropping from the surface of the mind, one sets one's biological clock to come back to complete awareness in about three minutes.

Step Three: *Approximately five minutes.*

After experiencing stillness, return to full consciousness at the surface of the mind and reflect on what one noticed about one's practice. Do not bolt into the day. The goal is to do this practice for ten minutes in the morning and evening to the best of one's ability and get into the experience of life.

Recommendation: Keep a journal to record experiences and progress. One may think one will remember everything, but many subtle gems of wisdom and growth will be forgotten.

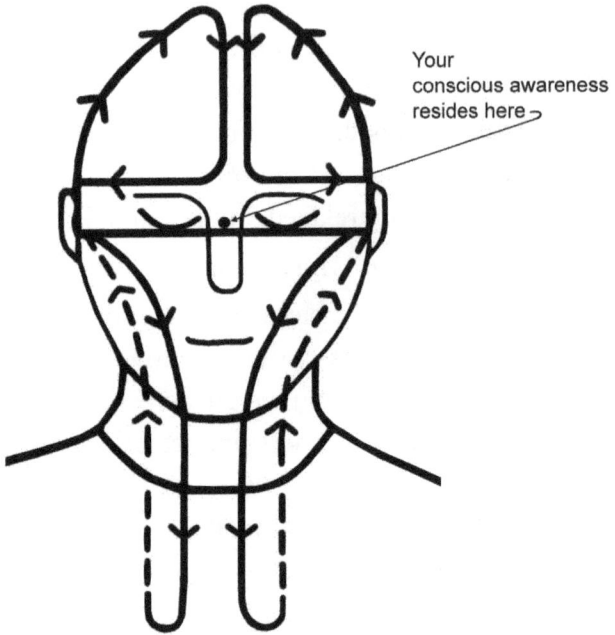

Your
conscious awareness
resides here

The Conscious Awareness

1. One's conscious awareness is who is reading this sentence right now.

2. The conscious awareness resides primarily at the surface of the mind, at eye level.

3. The conscious awareness is the liaison between the intellectual outside physical world and the inside world of emotion.

4. Where one directs one's attention is where the conscious awareness will be.

5. The conscious awareness can be directed outward, into the outer physical environment to heighten awareness of physical surroundings (i.e., sights, sounds, movement).

6. The conscious awareness can be directed inward, so that one becomes self-aware of one's inner world (i.e., thoughts, emotions, internalized fears).

7. The conscious awareness operates in three basic ways: mind function, brain function, and/or dysfunction.
   a. Mind function: associated with one's mental feeling sense or the observing part of us known as perception.
   b. Brain function: associated with the two physical hemispheres of the brain and the intellect. The conscious awareness can be directed into the brain/intellect to think (i.e., read, spell, perform mathematical equations, or analyze concepts) in the lesser Kelee region.
   c. Dysfunction: associated with misperception from compartments or negative "issues" (i.e., "baggage" or emotional "buttons") that are trapped in the Kelee.

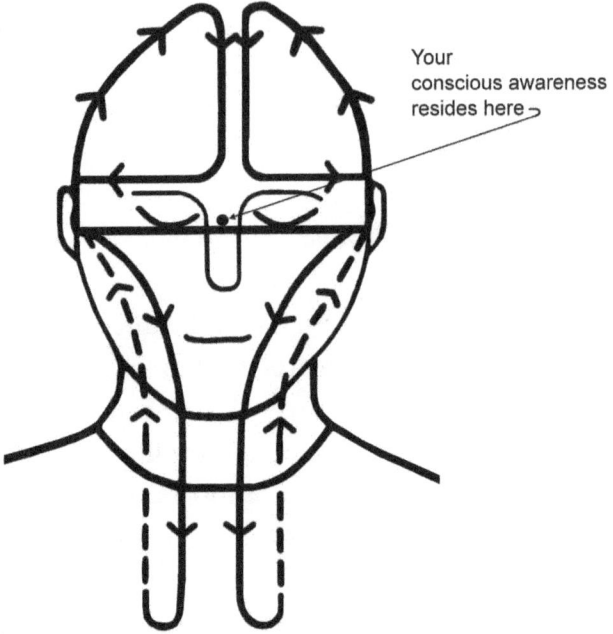

Your
conscious awareness
resides here

Brain Function and Mind Function

Brain Function Thinks and Analyzes

1. Brain function thinks, analyzes, stores data in the memory from existing knowledge in the intellect, runs the physical body, and is associated with the lesser Kelee region.
2. Brain function is associated with electrochemical physical energy.
3. The tendency in brain function is to rationalize, justify, defend, and control life.
4. If one is not able to mentally feel a relaxed conscious awareness, one will remain thinking in brain function.
5. One must be able to locate and feel the conscious awareness and allow it to relax and soften to begin the process of moving from brain function into mind function.
6. If one is not able to let go of the thinking or chatter from brain function, one will not enter into the calm, centered, deeper states of awareness experienced in mind function.

Mind Function Mentally Feels or Senses

1. Mind function mentally feels or senses as an objective observer and is synonymous with a relaxed feeling sense or clear perception. Mind function leads into deeper states of awareness and knowing associated with the greater Kelee region.
2. Mind function is a relaxed, fluid, subtle form of energy.
3. To master mind function, one must let go of the thinking in brain function and allow the conscious awareness to drop inside, below the surface of the mind, and open up to one's innate feeling sense found in the greater Kelee.

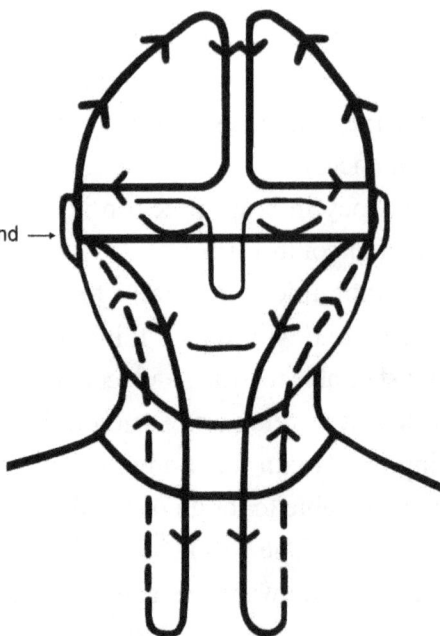

The surface of the mind ⟶
is at eye level

The Surface of the Mind

1. The surface of the mind is a division point between the lesser Kelee and the greater Kelee. The lesser Kelee is associated with the brain and the intellect. The greater Kelee is associated with emotion and deeper states of mind.

2. The surface of the mind is a flat plane of electrochemical energy at eye level.

3. By mentally feeling where one's thoughts are right now, one will feel them at eye level on the surface of the mind.

4. The surface of the mind serves as a reception point for incoming information, a point of contemplation, and a place to make decisions.

5. Thinking takes place on the surface of the mind. It is the work table of the mind.

6. The surface of the mind works best when cleared daily of distracting thoughts.

7. Unresolved thoughts left on the surface of the mind tend to make one think. Too many thoughts on the surface of the mind generate frustration, distraction, and fragmentation, thus potentially leading to the inability to focus.

8. Natural focus does not occur through a process of blocking out thought. It occurs when one has complete undistracted focus on one thought.

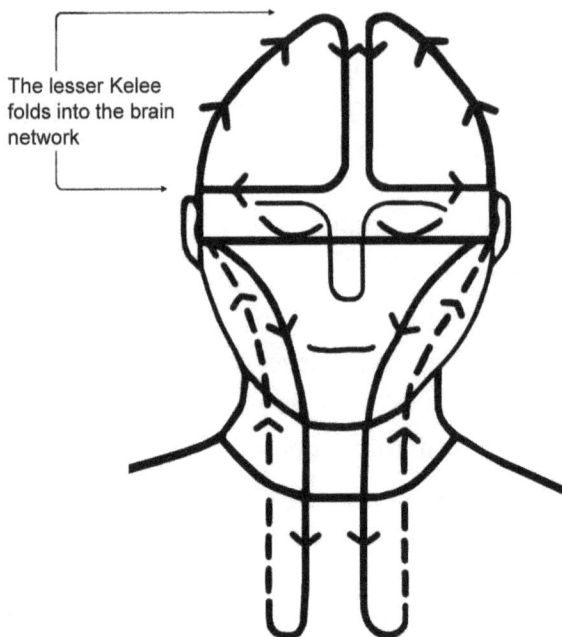

The lesser Kelee
folds into the brain
network

The Lesser Kelee

1. The energy of the lesser Kelee flows from the surface of the mind out laterally from the center, up over the top of the brain, then down in between both hemispheres of the brain, and folds into the brain network.

2. The lesser Kelee is associated with the brain, the intellect, and the thinking process.

3. The lesser Kelee region is analytical, based in linear time, and operates in a three-dimensional realm of height, width, and depth.

4. Compartments in the lesser Kelee region have to do with issues regarding the outside physical world—people, places, and things.

5. One's conscious awareness associated with the lesser Kelee region tends to create attachments to people and things in an attempt to be in control.

6. The most physically uncomfortable compartments in the lesser Kelee region are tension headaches, which are formed when one has either accepted or created intense negative emotion.

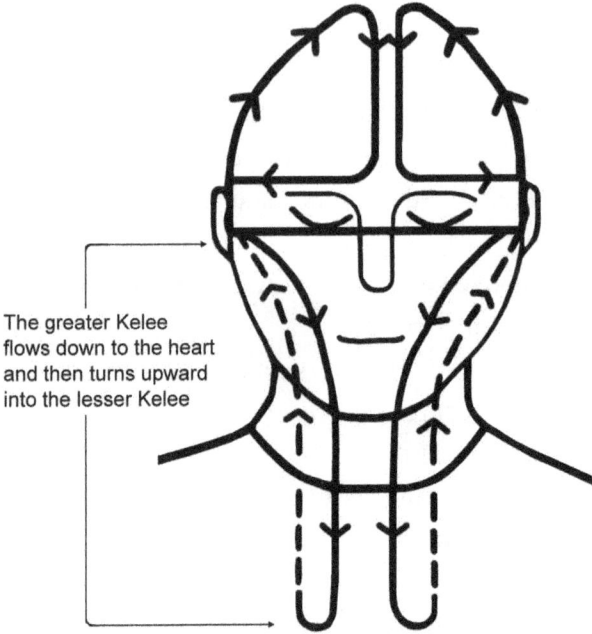

The greater Kelee
flows down to the heart
and then turns upward
into the lesser Kelee

The Greater Kelee

1. The energy of the greater Kelee flows from the surface of the mind, down to about where one's heart is and then turns upward to join in with the lesser Kelee.
2. The greater Kelee is associated with a feeling process, emotion, and matters of the heart.
3. The greater Kelee is nonlinear in nature and operates without an awareness of time.
4. The greater Kelee is where all emotion flows from as an expression of one's life.
5. Compartments in the greater Kelee have to do with how one feels about oneself.
6. Heartaches are the deepest of the human experience and are felt in the greater Kelee.
7. The greater Kelee is where one can move out of analytical thinking, and with practice, into pure perception of mind.
8. The greater Kelee is where one can learn to be completely still at one point.
9. The greater Kelee is infinite in nature.
10. The greater Kelee is where the emotions of love and contentment are realized and then experienced.

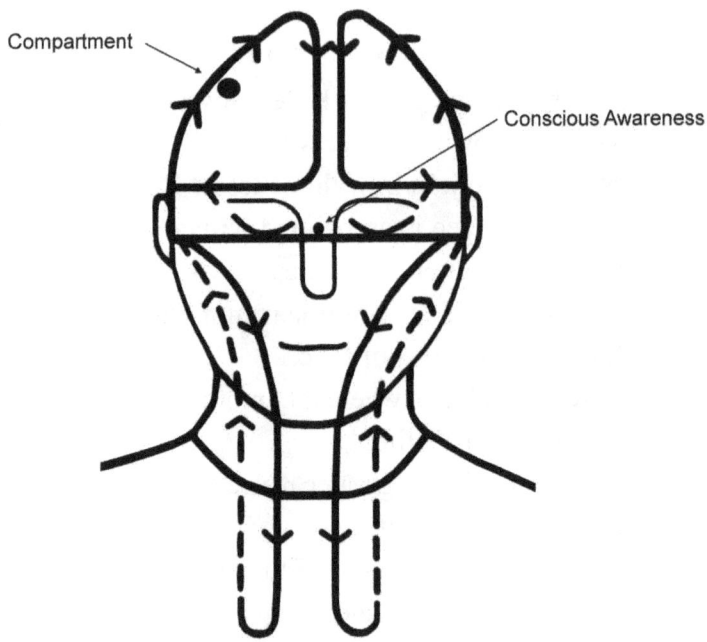

Compartment

Conscious Awareness

Compartments

1. Compartments are called many names in our society: "baggage," "issues," emotional "buttons," and dysfunction, to name a few.
2. From birth until this moment in time, energy from life experience is pouring through one's mind. When one, not knowing any better, takes in a negative experience, the thought can become trapped in the Kelee as a compartment.
3. Compartments form in two basic ways:

    a. When one internalizes a negative experience in an effort to control negativity.

    b. When one cannot face the harshness of reality and internally self-creates an illusion to offset discomfort.
4. Compartments can superimpose over the brain or form on the surface of the mind.
5. Compartments can exist in the lesser and greater Kelee.
6. There are two extreme forms of compartments:

    a. Anxiety-based.

    b. Depression-based.

    Both drain electrochemical energy from the immune system.
7. There are two basic ways compartments stay alive:

    a. By engaging oneself (e.g., being angry at oneself).

    b. By engaging another (e.g., being angry at another).
8. Compartments can exist in a conscious, subconscious, or unconscious form.

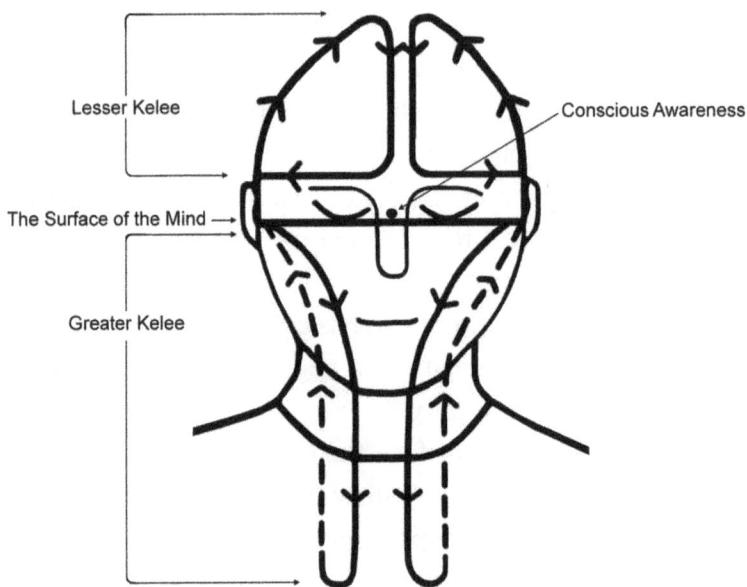

Lesser Kelee

Conscious Awareness

The Surface of the Mind →

Greater Kelee

Looping

1. Looping occurs when one's conscious awareness is attached to a negative compartment that circulates in a closed loop.
2. When a compartment is triggered by external stimuli, one's conscious awareness can cause a domino effect by initiating a loop of linked negative thoughts.
3. A closed loop of negativity between one's conscious awareness and a compartment will result in a constant stream of negative chattering thoughts.
4. Looping keeps one trapped in the past because all compartments are rooted in previous disharmonious experiences. This interferes with living openly to life's experience in the present moment.
5. One can loop with one's own compartments or with another person's compartments.

Cessation of Looping

1. The first step to stop looping is to know that it is occurring.
2. Looping is consciously diminished when one calms the electrochemical energy of brain function, thus weakening the energy that sustains looping.
3. Looping is further diminished when one's conscious awareness relaxes and does not engage with one's own compartments or another person's compartments.
4. Looping is broken when one learns to live detached in mind function instead of attached in brain function. Detachment is learned through doing Kelee meditation.

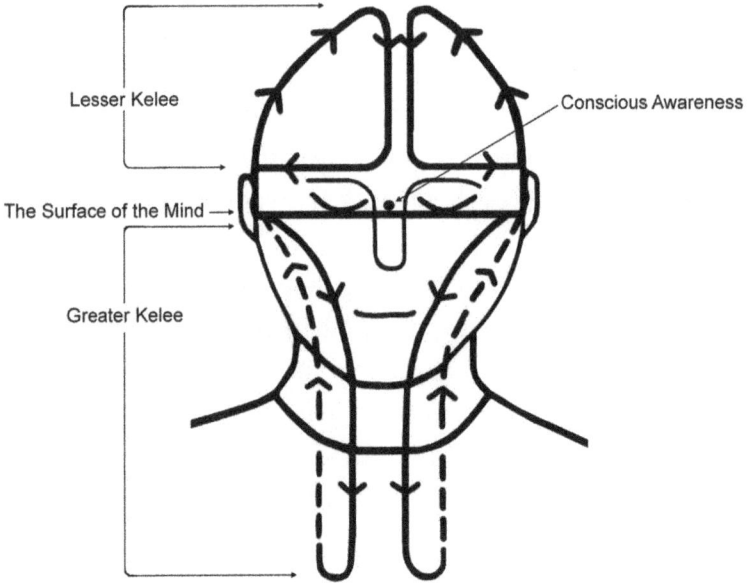

Lesser Kelee

Conscious Awareness

The Surface of the Mind

Greater Kelee

Detachment from Internal Compartments

1. Detachment refers to the state of being unaffected by negative emotion.
2. Detachment allows for dissolution of compartments because one becomes truly unaffected by negative thoughts and emotions associated with compartments.
3. When one attaches to people or things, dependencies are formed. This leads to emotional and/or physical pain/compartments when these attachments are broken.
4. Detachment allows one to operate without the conditioning of society and the limitation of time.
5. Detachment defines a truly open mind, and allows one to live freely by seeing life as it really is, and not how the outside world (i.e., media, advertising) would have one see life.
6. There are three basic steps to learn detachment:

    a. Mentally locate and feel one's conscious awareness and allow it to soften and relax. Relaxing one's conscious awareness through compartments in the lesser Kelee region dissolves them over time.

    b. Allow one's relaxed conscious awareness to open to the innate space found in the greater Kelee, and learn to be still at one point.

    c. When compartments are not electrochemically fed by conscious, subconscious, or unconscious negativity, they lose their energy and dissolve. When one lives in mind function, one will detach from compartments.
7. True detachment is freedom from pain. Detachment is a feeling of being connected to oneself and others, without the pain associated with attachment.

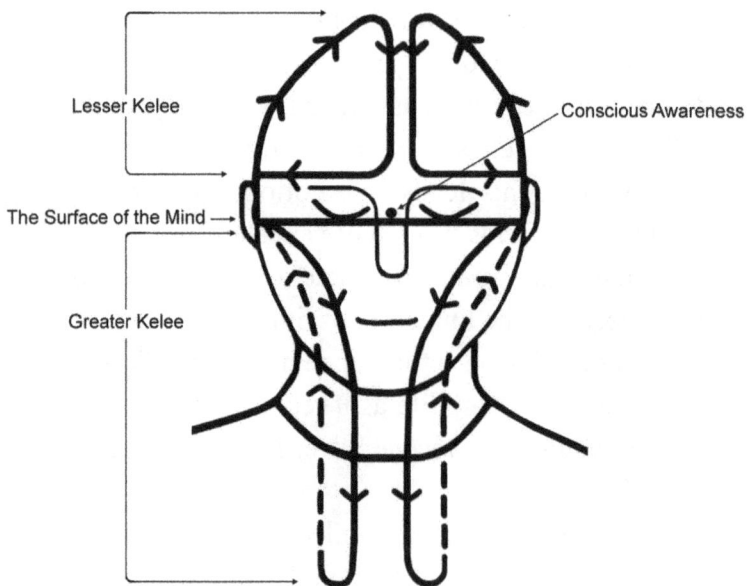

Lesser Kelee

Conscious Awareness

The Surface of the Mind

Greater Kelee

Processing of Compartments

1. Processing internal negative compartments begins when one's own mental resistance relaxes.
2. In order to avoid feeling the negativity of a compartment, most people block out issues by the self-creation of an electrochemical mental wall of resistance. In actuality, this technique reinforces and keeps compartments alive in one's Kelee. It is an illusion that one can permanently protect oneself from feeling one's compartments.
3. One may feel emotional discomfort or moodiness while processing; however, when the compartment passes, one will not experience the influence of that particular compartment again.
4. One may experience physiological effects when processing, such as low energy, headaches, nausea, depression, or anxiety. If a compartment was linked with physical discomfort at the time it formed, it will mimic the same response when it processes out. The physical discomfort will cease when the compartment is released.
5. When a compartment dissolves, it cannot be triggered again. Some compartments can appear similar, but upon close inspection they are not. One may have layers of similar types of compartments that are chronologically stacked in one's Kelee.
6. Processing is a sign that Kelee meditation is working correctly.

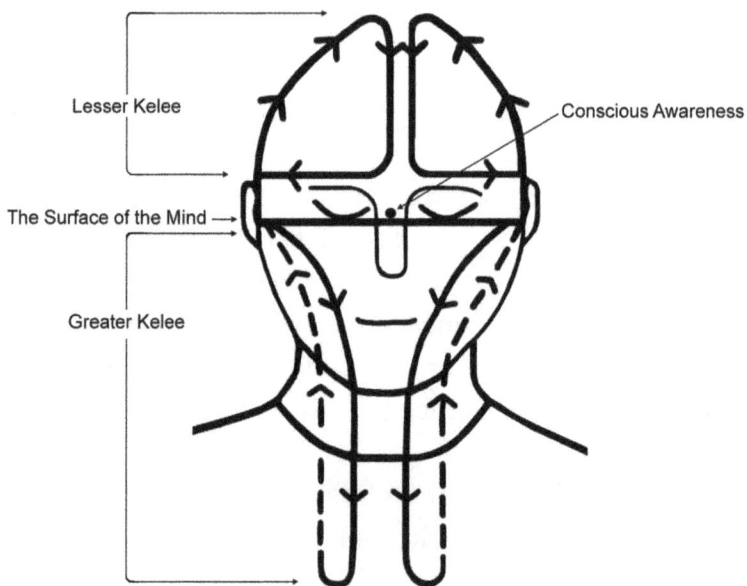

Lesser Kelee

Conscious Awareness

The Surface of the Mind

Greater Kelee

The Flow of the Kelee

1. Within the Kelee, the three-dimensional linear moment of time meets the non-linear moment of mental feeling and perception, bringing the two together at the surface of the mind.

2. The energy of the Kelee flows in upon itself, without beginning or end. Within the flow of the Kelee is a single point of perception known as the conscious awareness.

3. When one hears of the proverbial flow of life, this is when the energy of the lesser Kelee and greater Kelee flow together in harmony.

4. One can either loop through the memory of who one thinks one is, or flow with who one feels one is in this present moment.

5. When one is centered in one's conscious awareness, one can learn to flow with the harmonious energy of one's Kelee and be present in the moment.

6. To open to the flow of the Kelee one must learn how to end one's own internal struggle.

7. When one wants to end mental and physical disharmony, Kelee meditation will teach one how harmony of mind can heal emotional and physiological problems.

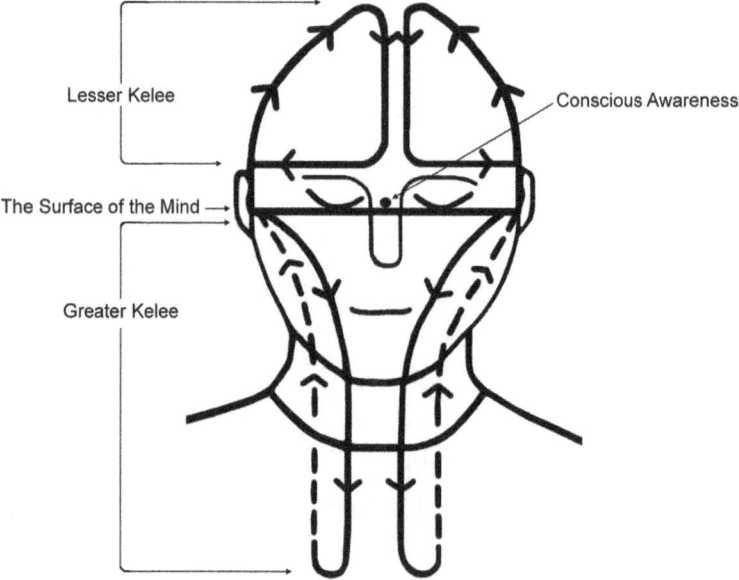

The Effects of Kelee Meditation

1. The effects of Kelee meditation will vary with each individual, depending on how diligent one is in doing this practice. Initially, the effects will be subtle in nature. However, over time the effects will be profound and will deepen with continued practice.

2. As one begins to practice Kelee meditation, one's mental thought activity will calm down. Calming down mentally will also relax tension in the physical body.

3. A signature of Kelee meditation is that experiences one used to react adversely to will no longer be an issue. When a compartment is dissolved, there is nothing to be triggered.

4. One's perception begins to open, thereby allowing more awareness of oneself and the world. One will notice and appreciate the beauty of nature—the details in life that one was too busy before to experience (i.e., the clouds in the sky, the wind blowing through the leaves in trees, the scent of flowers, and the singing of birds). As one learns to care for oneself, the people that one loves become more important than things or possessions.

5. Stress drops away and is replaced with a feeling of ease and contentment in one's life.

6. Psychologically, one feels better about oneself because there is less mental tension.

7. Physiologically, one feels better because one's mind is in harmony. Harmony promotes a stronger immune system, thus allowing the physical body to heal naturally.

These effects are just a few of the harmonious changes that will occur from doing Kelee meditation.

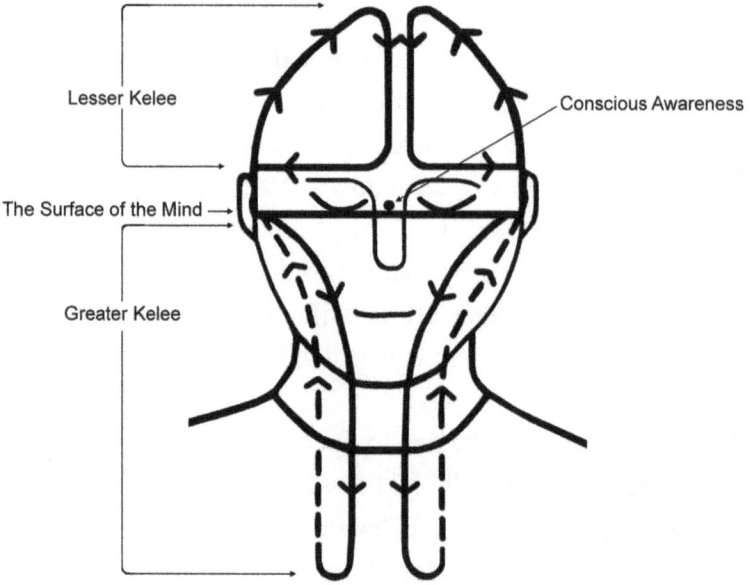

Lesser Kelee

Conscious Awareness

The Surface of the Mind →

Greater Kelee

Overview of Kelee Meditation

Step One

One locates and mentally feels one's conscious awareness at the top of the head. From the top of the head, one mentally relaxes one's conscious awareness into a flat plane of awareness. Allow this plane of awareness to soften and pass through both hemispheres of the brain, ultimately settling at the surface of the mind. When a thought or image distracts the conscious awareness, simply let it pass by. At the surface of the mind, one should be mentally calm and relaxed, but not actively thinking. When the relaxed horizontal plane of conscious awareness reaches the surface of the mind, one gently brings the conscious awareness to a single point of perception. Step One should take about two minutes.

Step Two

From a single point of perception, allow the conscious awareness to drop below the surface of the mind to a natural still point within the greater Kelee. Letting go of sense consciousness at the surface of the mind and experiencing total stillness within the greater Kelee is the goal of Step Two. Stillness is defined as a non-distracted, one-pointed awareness of self. It is achieved when there is an absence of thinking. If one is visualizing, trying to resolve an issue, planning activities, or distracted by the five physical senses while meditating, one is thinking and not doing this practice. After experiencing stillness, one returns to full consciousness at the surface of the mind. Step Two should end after about three minutes.

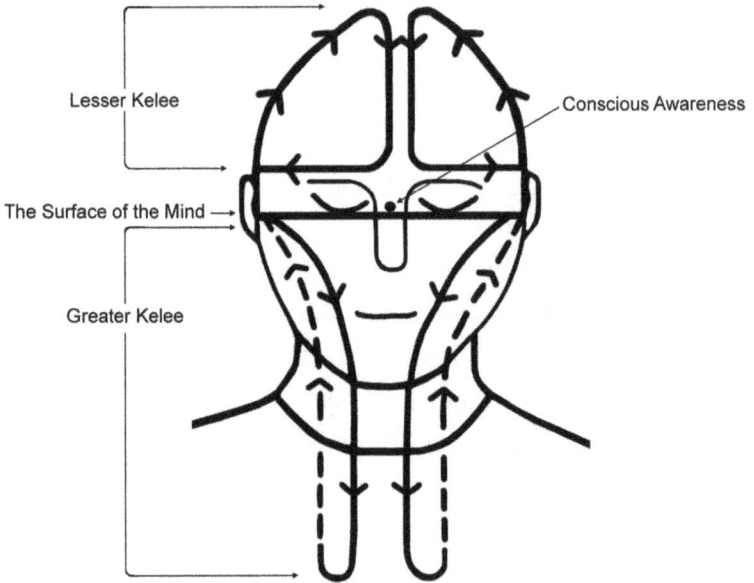

Lesser Kelee

Conscious Awareness

The Surface of the Mind →

Greater Kelee

Overview of Kelee Meditation (*continued*)

Step Three

Upon returning from meditation (stillness), one reflects on the quality of one's practice through introspection and contemplation.

Introspection is when one looks within one's Kelee from the surface of the mind and reflects on the quality of one's meditation. The introspection portion of Kelee meditation requires one to truthfully evaluate one's meditation and is for retrospective and observational purposes.

Contemplation is when one ponders one's observations. This provides an opportunity for self-understanding. The time devoted to contemplation will teach one a great deal about oneself. Questions to ask during contemplation:

1. Can I mentally feel my conscious awareness at the top of my head, relaxing down to the surface of my mind?
2. Was my mind busy with thought activity?
3. Did I feel myself drop into the greater Kelee with a sense of depth?
4. Does my mind and nervous system feel calmer?

It is difficult to completely still one's mind on command. The discipline of reaching stillness is an ongoing process. Excellence takes time. It is important that one is honest and kind when grading the quality of one's meditation. The quality of stillness will improve with time and practice. As long as one sincerely puts in the effort to help oneself, the results will come.

Step Three of Kelee meditation should be a minimum of five minutes.

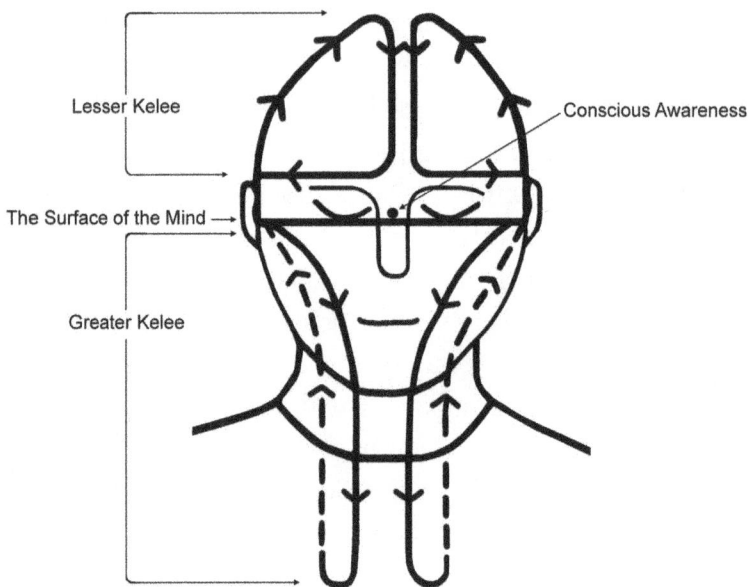

Lesser Kelee

Conscious Awareness

The Surface of the Mind →

Greater Kelee

Conceptual Medical Model
of Kelee Meditation

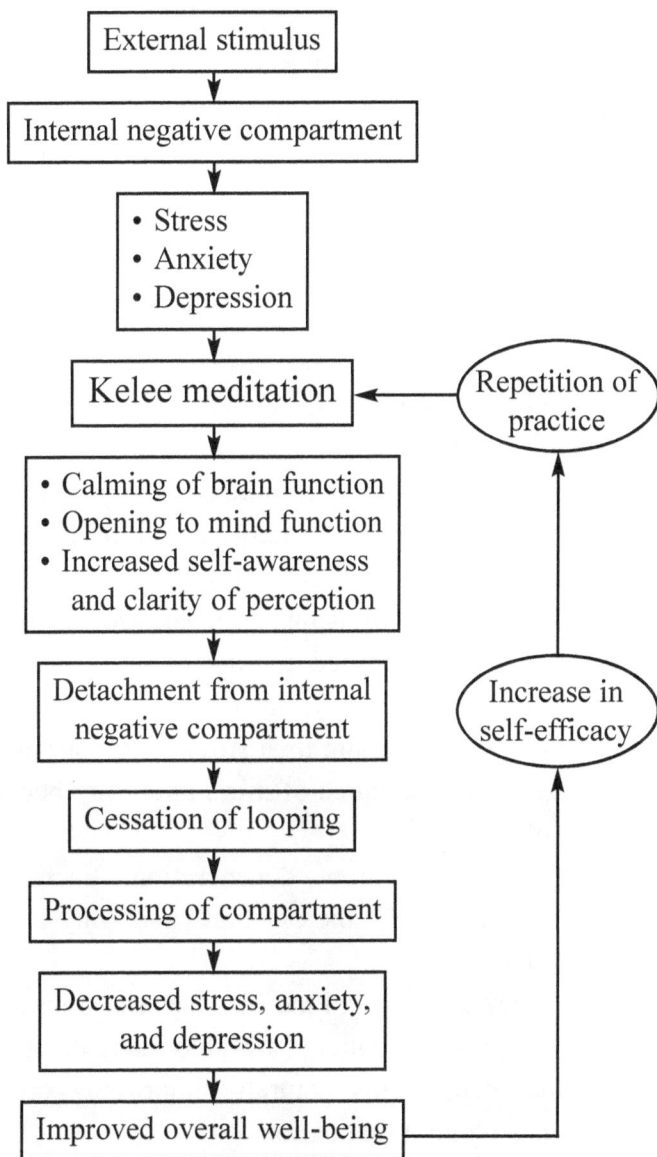

External stimulus

↓

Internal negative compartment

↓

- Stress
- Anxiety
- Depression

↓

Kelee meditation ← Repetition of practice

↓

- Calming of brain function
- Opening to mind function
- Increased self-awareness and clarity of perception

↓

Detachment from internal negative compartment

↓

Cessation of looping

↓

Processing of compartment

↓

Decreased stress, anxiety, and depression

↓

Improved overall well-being

Increase in self-efficacy

The Ins and Outs
of Kelee Meditation

1. A healthy physical body is supported by a healthy clear mind via Kelee meditation.

2. The side effects of Kelee meditation are actually benefits; a still mind balances the electrochemical of the physical body naturally.

3. One of the first observations you will notice is that things that used to bother you, no longer do. The first time this happens, you will be startled. You'll ask yourself, "Shouldn't that have affected me?" But it does not.

4. Another observation you will have is becoming aware of things you have not noticed before, such as the clouds in the sky, the many shades of green in the trees, birds and butterflies flying by, and the wind in your face. All of nature will become more vibrant.

5. The rewards received from Kelee meditation are experienced as a happy, unworried mind in your daily activities. Once again, total stillness in your practice is the goal, with balance of mind and body becoming a way of being.

6. Kelee meditation slows degeneration. Each time you still your mind, the mental and physical body rejuvenates.

7. Efficiency at work will increase because your conscious awareness is not scattered with too many thoughts from compartments. This naturally improves your ability to focus without distraction.

8. A deeper self-awareness enhances relationships at home and work, with the ability to give from the heart without expecting anything in return.

9. It is not unusual to feel a small drop in physical energy after beginning Kelee meditation, as you wean your mind off adrenaline-based, anxious energy. After a short period of time, your energy level will stabilize into an overall feeling of calmness and you will have a new understanding of stable electrochemical energy.

10. When you begin to drop the walls of resistance in your mind, you may feel some emotional discomfort as you process out compartments. Once a compartment is gone, you will not experience that particular dysfunction again.

11. Compartments affect the conscious awareness in three ways:

    a. Being consumed: when your conscious awareness is consumed by a compartment, and you are completely controlled by it and unaware of how the compartment is influencing your behavior.

    b. Being influenced: when your conscious awareness feels the compartment, but you are not controlled by it and you are aware of the compartment's influence.

    c. Being free: when your conscious awareness is unaffected by compartmentalization and you are totally aware of your freedom.

12. When you are processing, be good to yourself. You may want to sleep more than usual. This is normal. Give yourself a mental health day, if you can. If not, pace yourself throughout your day.

13. From time to time you will experience physiological effects when processing, such as headaches, nausea, low energy, depression, or anxiety. If a compartment was linked with physical discomfort at the time it was formed, it will mimic the same response when it is being processed out. Any physical discomfort will cease when the electrochemical compartment is dissolved.

14. Depression, worry, sadness, and all negative behavior toward oneself will eventually disappear altogether as you continue to practice Kelee meditation.

15. As negative, energy-draining compartments are deleted, the immune system is boosted and freed to function at optimal efficiency.

16. Elation occurs when the space occupied by dysfunction is replaced by the true nature of your being. Elation is a reward for your diligence and manifests as a potent, natural, euphoric feeling, thereby stimulating the release of endorphins and the body's natural tranquilizers.

17. If you are slow to wake up in the morning or too tired at bedtime, do Kelee meditation whenever possible; however, the goal is to become accustomed to a morning and evening routine. Sit with your spine erect when doing Kelee meditation. Do not do Kelee meditation lying down; it is too easy to go to sleep. Stillness of mind is not sleep!

18. If you are falling asleep while meditating, you are either too tired or too relaxed. When your conscious awareness is too relaxed, it will spread out and wander. Refocus by pulling all of your awareness to a pinpoint within you.

The sleep/stillness line of distinction takes time to master. Do Kelee meditation to the best of your ability and consider it a success because you did it.

19. Set your biological clock for about three minutes before you drop into your greater Kelee. This becomes automatic after the first few times.

20. The time you are in your Kelee is not the time to investigate what you see and experience! If you are thinking or drifting off, your conscious awareness cannot be still. The absence of thought-form images allows stillness to occur and is the objective of Kelee meditation.

21. Keep a journal to record your experience after your practice. This will be a record of your personal growth and development.

22. Do Kelee meditation even when you do not feel like it; this is when you need to do it the most.

23. Once you find your conscious awareness, the surface of the mind, the lesser and greater Kelee, you will have found a way to understand the mystery of thought and emotion and its effects on your mind and body.

24. The three disciplines of Kelee meditation are Meditation, Introspection, and Contemplation.

25. The three P's of Kelee meditation are Practice, Persistence, and Patience.

26. Do Kelee meditation for ten minutes in the morning and ten minutes in the evening.

27. If you have not given Kelee meditation at least six months, you have not really given yourself a chance to know what a clear mind feels like.

Never underestimate the power of calmness to start the process of health and regeneration. Stress does not allow the nervous system to work properly. It is calmness of mind that soothes the physical body into healing. To heal, we must calm ourselves and allow ourselves to be peaceful. For all those who are looking to heal from the inside out, a quote from my first book *The Way is Within* is appropriate.

"Be at peace with yourself.
If you are not at peace with yourself,
you are at peace with nothing."

—*Ron W. Rathbun*

About the Author

Ron W. Rathbun's fascination with human emotions and the mind stems back to his teenage years. Ron was enrolled at a community college to begin studying psychology when he met Dr. Eugene C. Larr, a retired professor from Cal Tech in Pasadena, California, who had two PhDs and three master's degrees. After meeting this man, Ron knew he had found his teacher—the one who would become his mentor. Ron studied and consulted privately with his mentor about the inner workings of the Kelee for twenty-eight years, until Dr. Larr's death in 2006.

Ron's career as a teacher began in 1985 and in January of 1993, he began teaching Kelee meditation. He has taught Kelee meditation to people from all walks of life, many of whom are physicians. In September of 2008, The University of California, San Diego Institutional Review Board granted full approval to begin a medical study to measure the change and effects of Kelee meditation on patients suffering from stress, anxiety and depression.

Ron Rathbun continues to research and study the effects of the mind on the immune system and nervous system in relation to healing the physiology of the body. Ron is an award-winning author of three books, *The Way is Within, The Silent Miracle,* and *The Kelee.* He is founder and president of the Kelee Foundation in Oceanside, California. Ron's teachings are centered in the thought that, *When the mind is brought into harmony, it will heal the physical body.*

Contact Us

What each person brings to the world is what they have within. It is our mission to offer, to all those who are seeking, a way to internally heal one's own mind through Kelee meditation. For it is the condition of one's Kelee that influences one's emotional and physical health and wellness.

The Kelee Foundation is a 501(c)(3) nonprofit, tax-exempt organization. It is generously funded by the donations of its loyal students and all those who recognize the health benefits of a clear mind. Please feel free to contact us if you are interested in learning more at www.thekelee.org.